MEDICAL
TERMINOLOGY

FOR HEALTH PROFESSIONALS

2024 - 2025

The Ultimate Guide to Effortlessly
Learn, Pronounce, and Grasp Medical
Terms in 30 Days

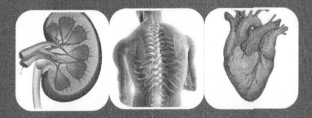

KAREN ANDERSSON
G. Meloni M.D.
DR MICHELLE SMILEY

Medical Terminology for Health Professionals 2024-2025

The Ultimate Guide to Effortlessly Learn, Pronounce, and Grasp Medical Terms in 30 Days

Karen Andersson
G. Meloni M.D.
Dr   Michelle Smiley

DISCLAIMER

Copyright © 2023 by Karen Andersson

Dedication

To all the aspiring healthcare professionals, curious minds, and learners embarking on the journey of mastering the intricate language of medicine,

This book is dedicated to you, the diligent seekers of knowledge. With unwavering commitment and passion, you've ventured into the world of Medical Terminology. Your pursuit of understanding the complex and multifaceted language of healthcare is both admirable and inspiring.

In these pages, you will find the keys to unlock the door to medical understanding. Our journey together begins with the basics and takes you through the intricate web of medical terms. From the significance of medical tests to the origins of these terms, from body systems to the creation of plurals – we cover it all.

In the pursuit of your noble calling, may this guide serve as your trusted companion. As you turn these pages, may you effortlessly learn, pronounce, and grasp medical terms within 30 days.

With the deepest respect for your commitment to this field, we embark on this educational voyage together. This book is dedicated to your relentless pursuit of knowledge and your desire to make a difference in the world of healthcare.

Wishing you a successful and fulfilling journey through "Medical Terminology for Beginners 2023-2024: The Ultimate Guide to Effortlessly Learn, Pronounce, and Grasp Medical Terms in 30 Days."

Sincerely,
Karen Andersson.

Table of contents

Final Thought

Introduction

Welcome and congratulations on acquiring the book "Medical Terminology Guide for Beginners." The field of medicine is incredibly expansive, filled with numerous terms and methods employed by medical experts. For those embarking on their medical journey without prior experience, deciphering these terms can be a daunting task.

Medical terminology serves as the universal language in the healthcare industry, encompassing human anatomy, physiology, clinical diagnoses, procedures, and processes. This language facilitates effective communication among medical professionals, allowing them to convey complex information concisely. Therefore, it's imperative for every healthcare professional to hone their understanding of medical terminology.

Medical science doesn't solely consist of complex jargon; it also features a multitude of straightforward terms that are accessible to all. Familiarizing yourself with these fundamental terms is key to grasping the core language of medicine. Equipping yourself with this foundational knowledge is invaluable for comprehending various medical examinations and reports that may pertain to you or your loved ones. It empowers you to decipher diagnostic reports and gain firsthand insights into your health, enabling you to make informed decisions.

The purpose of this book is to demystify the diverse terminology found in medical reports. Throughout your life, you'll encounter a multitude of examinations, each accompanied by terminology that might initially seem perplexing. We are here to provide you with guidance to enrich your overall knowledge, thereby enhancing your capacity to navigate the world of healthcare.

Inside this book, you will discover extensive alphabetical lists of root words, prefixes, and suffixes, along with explanations. Additionally, we delve into terminology specific to various parts of the body and body systems. You'll learn how to break down a medical term and unveil its meaning, as well as how to pluralize terms and more.

This manual will assist you in:

Grasping the meaning of medical terminology. Understanding, spelling, and composing medical terms for effective communication and documentation in healthcare.

Explaining the significance of medical terms to others.

Deconstructing intricate words and utilizing their components to decipher and establish the meanings of medical terminology.

Applying the prefixes, root words, combining forms, and suffixes learned in this guide to construct medical terms.

A person with a strong grasp of medical vocabulary is fortunate, especially for those involved in medical fields, as they frequently employ scientific terminology. Some commonly used medical terms in everyday language include arthritis, hepatitis, or leukemia, while others are acknowledged as more intricate. This guide will equip you to become proficient, enabling you to decode unfamiliar and complex terms and comprehend them thoroughly.

So, let's embark on the journey of simplifying medical terminology!

Chapter 1

The Significance of Medical Tests and Medication

Before delving into the intricacies of medical terminology to provide you with a clear understanding of various terms, it's essential to grasp some key details. Understanding the importance of medical tests and the reasons people opt for such assessments and medications will enhance your comprehension of the subject.

1. *Prioritizing Your Health*

First and foremost, it's crucial to recognize that nothing surpasses the importance of your health. Sometimes, the state of your health may deteriorate unnoticed. Medical tests and examinations are your window to a comprehensive understanding of your true health condition. Regular medical check-ups play a pivotal role in enabling you to gauge your overall well-being. There is no room for complacency when it comes to your health, so it's imperative to discuss your test results with your healthcare provider and seek clarification on any aspects that may appear unclear.

2. *Enhanced Medical Guidance*

When your physician recommends a range of medical examinations, it eliminates guesswork and ensures that you receive appropriate medical assistance when necessary. Many individuals tend to postpone medical assessments, placing their health on the backburner. However, it's crucial to acknowledge that these tests serve a purpose. They reveal the true state of your health, guiding you toward the most suitable course of treatment. Being informed about your health is far more advantageous than ignoring your doctor's recommendations for regular check-ups.

3. *The Benefits of Routine Check-ups*

You don't have to wait until you are ill or experiencing health complications to undergo health check-ups. Ideally, it should become a routine practice to schedule periodic check-ups. This practice is valuable because it allows you to detect potential issues in advance. Regular check-ups serve as a proactive approach to identify and address potential health concerns before they become more serious.

In today's fast-paced world, where people are constantly occupied with various activities, it can be challenging to gain a clear understanding of one's well-being. Additionally, many medical conditions may remain silent for extended periods before displaying any symptoms. Therefore, it becomes essential to prioritize routine check-ups at regular intervals. This proactive methodology can have a tremendous effect. For instance, early detection of conditions like breast cancer can significantly impact the prognosis.

4. *Cost Savings in Healthcare*

We are well aware of the financial burden associated with purchasing medications and covering medical expenses. Healthcare costs and medical bills can often become overwhelming. In such situations, opting for medical tests and early diagnosis can lead to substantial cost savings in the long run. The escalating cost of healthcare is a reality, and if timely check-ups are neglected, it could result in leaving illnesses undetected until they reach a critical stage – a situation that's far from ideal.

These are some of the crucial aspects that underscore the importance of medical tests and examinations. It's imperative to heed these considerations. Medical exams not only safeguard your well-being but also contribute to improved health. Therefore, it is advisable to undergo these assessments when they are due or as recommended by your healthcare provider. Now that you understand their significance, let's shift our focus to exploring the key terminologies and language you may encounter.

Chapter 2

Introduction to General Medical Terminology

In this chapter, we delve into the world of numerous diseases that affect millions of individuals. Understanding our bodies is crucial, and thus, we begin with the fundamentals. Let's explore basic medical tests and, in the following chapter, different types of medications.

What's Covered?

When we discuss essential medical terminology, we'll address various key aspects, including:

- Abbreviations for diagnostic tests like ECF, EEG, MRI, CT scans, and more.
- Common illnesses that affect many people.
- Health insurance-related terminologies.
- Medical equipment for conducting tests, such as BPM.
- Hospital departments.
- Abbreviations used in hospital settings.

- Basic medical terms.
- Categories and types of prescribed medicines.
- An introduction to basic human anatomy.

This list isn't exhaustive, as there's much more to explore. If you're not from a medical background, it may take time to grasp all these terms. Gradually building your knowledge base will improve your understanding of this important topic.

Body Systems

Now, let's examine the core systems within your body for a better understanding of which medicines are intended for specific body parts. This knowledge is foundational.

The Skeletal System: This comprises the body's structural framework, including bones, axial skeleton, and joints.

The Muscular System: Connecting bones, muscles are present throughout the body and are essential for various activities.

The Respiratory System: Focused on breathing, it encompasses body parts like the neck, pharynx, trachea, lungs, larynx, and bronchi.

The Endocrine System: Concerned with hormones, it includes the thyroid, pancreas, adrenal glands, gonads, and the pituitary gland.

The Nervous System: Often referred to as the central nervous system, it coordinates and controls the functions of other systems. This system includes the brain, spinal cord, and sensitive nerves and organs.

The Cardiovascular System: Comprising the heart, blood, and blood vessels, this system is responsible for pumping blood.

The Reproductive System: Focused on reproduction, it involves the genital organs of both males and females.

The Urinary System

This system encompasses various vital organs, including the kidneys, bladder, urethra, ureter, and more. These organs collaborate to filter waste from your body, purify your blood, and regulate the balance of water and salt within your system as impurities are removed.

The Immune System

Among the body's most essential systems, the immune system is responsible for maintaining the body's health and defending against various diseases. It comprises multiple components that protect the body from foreign invaders by releasing antibodies into the bloodstream, aiding in the fight against illness.

The Auditory and Ocular System

The auditory and ocular systems are often discussed together since they are part of the sensory organ system. This system includes the eyes, auditory organs, glands, and various bones and muscles that facilitate vision and hearing.

These are some of the primary systems in the body, and any medical ailment typically affects one or more of these systems. Numerous tests are available to assess the functionality of these anatomical components.

Anatomical Planes

Understanding the human body involves recognizing its various positions and planes. Similar to peeling the layers of an onion, gaining insights into your anatomy requires knowledge of anatomical positions and planes. For instance, how would you identify discomfort in the heart region without understanding its anatomical location? Familiarity with these terms is invaluable when visiting a hospital or diagnostic center. They provide crucial information for diagnosis and enable you to interpret results. Here's a key term to remember:

Anterior: This term denotes the front-facing part of the body.

Deep: Refers to the portion of the body situated closer to its core or center.

Lateral: Describes a plane that is positioned toward the side of the body.

Distal: Signifies a part that is distant from the specified reference point.

Posterior: Denotes the plane consisting of the body's back.

Superficial: Indicates the portion closer to the body's surface.

Note: Incorrectly using any of these planes in a sentence can significantly alter its meaning. When defining something, always be specific about the anatomical plane you are referring to.

Now, moving on to the topic of **MEMBRANES**

An understanding of the five types of *membranes* in the human body is crucial for enhancing your grasp of medical terminology.
These membranes line internal organs and constitute a significant portion of human anatomy.

A disruption in any of these membranes can lead to severe harm, potentially preventing unexpected organ or tube ruptures.
Expanding your knowledge about different membrane types will empower you to comprehend your diagnosis and communicate with your healthcare provider more effectively.

Let's delve into the five major types of membranes in the body:

Meninges: Comprising three interconnected tissue membranes, these are located between the spinal cord and the brain, providing protective coverage for these vital organs.

Mucous Membrane: Found on the interior walls of organs and lining various tubes, this membrane safeguards the respiratory, digestive, reproductive, and urinary systems from wear and tear.

Synovial Membrane: Composed of diverse connective tissues, these membranes line joint cavities, playing a crucial role in facilitating bone movement by lubricating the joint spaces.

Serous Membrane: This vital membrane can be found throughout your body, lining various cavities to shield them from potential ruptures and safeguarding internal organs like your heart.

Cutaneous Membrane: The largest and most significant membrane in your body is the cutaneous membrane, which covers your entire skeletal framework - your skin.

After acquiring essential knowledge about these membranes, you will gain a deeper understanding of your body. Whether you receive a prescription or are asked to undergo tests, these actions primarily aim to address issues within your bodily systems. Later, we will also explore different categories of medicine, which will help you discern the general conditions your doctor is treating.

In the realm of medical science, the key is to adopt a systematic approach. It's crucial to follow a structured method rather than attempting to grasp a multitude of concepts simultaneously. If you have any doubts about what's being discussed, don't hesitate to ask your physician the necessary questions.

Initially, delving into the world of biology and medical science can be overwhelming, especially for those not inherently interested in these fields or unfamiliar with human anatomy. The amount of information to absorb and explore can be substantial.

However, this shouldn't discourage you, as you never know when a bit of medical knowledge might be invaluable. Sometimes, having the right information can make a significant difference and even save someone's life. Therefore, it's essential to expand your own understanding in the field of medicine. Additionally, taking a first aid course can further enhance your comprehension of common ailments.

Chapter 3

Exploring the Diverse Realm of Medicines

In the world of medicine, an array of broad categories exists to classify these indispensable remedies. Although it is challenging to encapsulate all medicines within specific categories, let's delve into these overarching classifications to shed light on their significance.

Sedatives: These medications are primarily enriched with sleep-inducing compounds, aiming to induce drowsiness when taken as prescribed. Sedatives play a multifaceted role, extending beyond just sleep aids. They often form an integral part of pain management, offering respite from short-term discomfort.

Antibiotics: Among the most frequently employed medicinal forms, antibiotics are crucial in combating bacterial infections that infiltrate the body. Typically, antibiotics are administered during common illnesses accompanied by fever to bolster the body's defense mechanisms and facilitate recovery.

Analgesics: These medications predominantly serve as pain relievers. The choice of analgesic and its dosage depends on the nature and intensity of pain, a determination best made by your healthcare provider. It's essential to exercise caution, as excessive use of analgesics can lead to adverse effects. Always seek the recommendation of a licensed medical professional before their usage and peruse the accompanying literature for contraindications.

Mineral and Vitamin Supplements: Medicines often incorporate vitamin and mineral tablets to address deficiencies in the body. Vitamin deficiencies are prevalent in many individuals. Identifying the specific deficiency through blood tests is essential. Once identified, you can opt for suitable supplements. Ideally, these supplements should be side effect-free, but it's prudent to consult with a healthcare expert before use.

Vaccines: While vaccines are typically administered through injections, they form a vital part of miscellaneous medicines. A myriad of vaccines has been developed to combat various health issues. Some vaccines are recommended during infancy, such as those for polio and chickenpox.

Growth Promoters: These are akin to vitamin supplements but cater to specific growth-related concerns. Growth can be stunted due to various factors, and these promoters aid in addressing the underlying issues. They should never be used without medical guidance.

These are the primary categories of medicines that provide a foundation for your understanding. Under each of these categories, numerous sub-categories exist. The right medication can help you navigate diverse health challenges, enhancing the prospects of a smooth and complete recovery. Medications may share similar compounds and benefits, but their prescription should always be entrusted to a medical professional rather than self-diagnosis.

Now that you've acquainted yourself with these main categories of medicines, let's embark on a journey to explore the intricacies of some of the most commonly used medical terms. Remember, take your time to absorb and gradually build your knowledge, as learning too much at once may prove overwhelming.

27

Chapter 4

Understanding the Origins of Medical Terms

Before diving into the world of medical terminology, it's crucial to master the art of decoding words and uncovering their core components. This process involves identifying the root or organic word, which serves as the foundation for understanding a term's true meaning. By honing this technique, you'll gain the ability to comprehend the essence of every medical term and how it has evolved over time.

You'll soon discover that each medical term holds its own unique story. Many English words have roots in the Greek or Latin languages, and by studying their prefixes and suffixes, you can unveil their precise meanings. Like any language, etymology serves as a valuable tool to dissect words into parts and retain this knowledge for versatile use, thanks to its general rules.

By mastering three fundamental components of any word, you'll unlock valuable insights into its organic meaning and how you can manipulate it to convey nuanced concepts:

Root Word: This is the core essence of a term, serving as the word's foundation. It is often combined with prefixes and suffixes to derive its exact meaning.

Prefixes: These elements are positioned at the beginning of a word, before the root word. Prefixes play a crucial role in conveying specific conditions or circumstances that enhance the word's meaning.

Suffixes: Found after the root word, suffixes are usually connected to the root word through a combining vowel. They provide information about a particular aspect of the body, especially in medical contexts, where they can indicate procedures, diseases, or specific conditions.

Additionally, you should become familiar with combining vowels and combining forms. When a vowel is used to link a root word to another root word or a suffix, it's referred to as a combining vowel. In medical terminology, "o" is the most commonly used combining vowel. A combining form, on the other hand, is a combination of the root word and the combining vowel.

Deconstructing Medical Terms

Now that you understand how words can be broken down into distinct parts, you can easily decode nearly any medical term. While it may require some practice and an initial understanding of root words, you can follow this pattern to deconstruct a word effectively:

Start at the end and identify the suffix in the word. Determine the meaning of the suffix.

Move to the beginning of the word and search for a prefix (not all words have one).

Decode the meaning of the prefix.

After removing the suffix and prefix, the root word will remain; identify it and unveil its meaning.

Combine all the identified meanings to form a comprehensive understanding.

Let's illustrate this process with an example:

"Cardiomyopathy." Starting from the end, you can recognize the suffix as "pathy," which is a common medical term indicating a disease or illness. The prefix here is "cardio," signifying anything related to the heart, with "o" serving as the combining vowel. The root word is "my/o," representing muscles. Therefore, "Cardiomyopathy" translates to a heart muscle disease.

Now, let's tackle a more complex example:

"Rhinorrhea." This word breaks down into two parts - "rrhea" and "Rhin/o." Beginning at the end, "rrhea" indicates a discharge or flow. Since there is no prefix in this word, we focus on the root word "rhin" (meaning nose) and the combining vowel "o." Thus, "Rhinorrhea" refers to a flow or discharge from the nose, simply put, a runny nose.

Understanding these concepts will empower you to decode medical terms with ease. To further assist you, we've compiled a list of commonly used root words, prefixes, and suffixes that will simplify your journey in understanding medical terminology. Dedicate yourself to learning this list diligently.

Root Words

In the realm of medical science, there exists a set of foundational words that are extensively used. When dissecting a word, you might encounter instances where a single term contains multiple root words. Here's a list of some of these essential root words:

- Hem or Hemat: Referring to blood or things related to blood.
- Chrom: Associated with color.
- Cephal: Pertaining to the head.
- Enter: Related to the intestine.
- Oste: Concerning bones.
- Vas: Denoting ducts or vessels.
- Synov: Relating to synovial joints, fluids, or membranes.
- Gastr: Connected to the stomach.
- Derm: Involving the skin.
- Phleb: Relating to veins.
- Thromb: Signifying a clot.
- My: Referring to muscles or things muscular.
- Onych: Linked to nails.
- Pulm: Connected to the lungs.
- Col: Concerning the colon.
- Aden: Pertaining to glands.
- Bio: Relating to life.
- Brachi: Associated with the arms.
- Anter: Referring to the front.
- Audi: Involving hearing.

- Abdomin: Connected to the abdomen.
- Cyt: Concerning cells.
- Bronch: Relating to bronchi.
- Carcin: Signifying cancer.
- Hist: Involving tissues.
- Gynec: Pertaining to females.
- Encephal: Related to the brain.
- Dors: Denoting the back.
- Or: Connected to the mouth.
- Optic: Signifying sight or matters related to vision.
- Ocul: Involving the eye.
- Lapar: Concerning the abdomen.
- Neur: Related to neurons or nerves.
- Ot: Pertaining to the ear or hearing.
- Path: Signifying disease or illness.
- Sept: Relating to infection.
- Pulmon: Connected to the lungs or respiratory matters.
- Pharmac: Involving drugs.
- Thyr: Pertaining to the thyroid gland.
- Trich: Signifying hairlike structures or hair.
- Thorac: Associated with the chest.
- Ventr: Referring to the frontal part of the body.
- Viscer: Denoting the internal organs of the body.

Prefixes

Identifying prefixes can sometimes be a bit challenging. Keep an eye out for these common prefixes that serve to enhance the meaning of root words by adding details like number, location, or time:

- Ec: Indicating something is outside.
- Ect: Referring to things outside.
- A: Signifying the absence of or something without.
- Peri: Denoting the surrounding area.
- End: Signifying something is within or inside.
- Poly: Referring to a multitude or many.
- Ab: Signifying something is away.
- Mon: Indicating one or single.
- Supra: Above something.
- Ad: Signifying something is nearby or adjacent.
- Trans: Referring to moving through, across, or crossing something.
- Ante: Signifying before or prior to something.
- Post: Indicating something is after or behind something.

Suffixes

As previously mentioned, suffixes are attached at the end of words and typically represent a condition, disorder, or illness. Here are some commonly used suffixes:

- Emia: Involving blood.
- Uria: Relating to urine or urination.
- Algia: Signifying pain or a sense of discomfort.
- Tripsy: Denoting crushing.
- Centesis: Referring to tapping or puncturing.
- Sclerosis: Indicating the hardening of something.
- Desis: Signifying the fusion or binding of two units.
- Plasty: Involving surgery, repair, or the plastic reconstruction of something.
- Ectomy: Pertaining to the surgical removal of something.
- Pexy: Denoting the surgical fixation of a unit or an organ.
- Graphy: Signifying recording.

By understanding and applying these root words, prefixes, and suffixes, you can easily decipher the meaning of most medical terms. All you need to do is break them down into their various components and reassemble them to unveil the word's meaning. While it may appear complex initially, with consistent practice, you'll become proficient in no time. So, grab your medical dictionary and embark on your journey to become a wordsmith in the medical field.

Chapter 5

Exploring Essential Medical Vocabulary

Now, let's delve into fundamental medical terminology that will enhance your comprehension. You might already be familiar with some of these terms, but there's always room for a refresher. Let's get started!

Acidosis
Description: This condition occurs when the blood has an excessive level of acid, often due to lung dysfunction reducing oxygen supply to the body.

Acute Myocardial Infarction (Heart Attack)
Description: Informally known as a heart attack, this condition arises from a sudden blockage in the main arteries supplying the heart, resulting in damage to heart muscles.

Addiction
Description: Addiction refers to excessive dependence on a substance, not limited to drugs, indicating a body's reliance on the specific substance.

Anemia
Description: Anemia is a medical condition marked by a decreased concentration of red blood cells in the blood, often leading to pale skin color.

Ancillary Services
Description: This term encompasses a wide range of services offered by healthcare facilities, beyond food and accommodation, such as surgical procedures, laboratory tests, and therapy.

Angina
Description: Angina refers to sharp cardiac pain caused by insufficient blood supply to the heart muscles, sometimes reaching severe levels and posing potential danger.

Anorexia
Description: Anorexia represents a loss of appetite, which can lead to physical and psychological issues when prolonged.

Antidepressant
Description: These medications are used to assist individuals in managing depression, enabling them to confront life's challenges.

Antiemetic
Description: Antiemetics are drugs administered to control vomiting.

Antipsychotic
Description: These drugs are utilized to treat individuals with psychosis, helping them return to a more stable mental state.

Apnea
Description: Apnea signifies a temporary pause in breathing, with Apnea of prematurity occurring in premature babies due to underdeveloped respiratory control.

Appendicitis
Description: Appendicitis arises when the appendix becomes inflamed, potentially causing pain, swelling, and infection, often necessitating surgical removal.

Arthritis

Description: Arthritis involves inflammation of the joints, often leading to pain and mobility issues, requiring appropriate evaluation and treatment.

Asthma
Description: Asthma is a lung disease triggered by various factors, commonly involving allergic reactions, leading to coughing and breathing difficulties.

Asphyxia
Description: Asphyxia occurs when there is an imbalance of oxygen and carbon dioxide in the body.

Acquired immune Deficiency Syndrome (AIDS)
Description: AIDS signifies a severe immune system failure, making it challenging for the body to resist bacterial and viral infections.

Bacteria
Description: Bacteria are microscopic organisms responsible for various human illnesses, often challenging to control due to their rapid reproduction.

Beneficiary

Description: The beneficiary is the person covered by health insurance who can receive benefits from the insurance company.

Benign
Description: Benign is used to describe a non-cancerous tumor.

Bilirubin
Description: Bilirubin is the yellow pigment in the blood that can cause skin to appear a prominent cream color when present in high levels.

Blood Count
Description: Blood count measures the quantity of white blood cells, red blood cells, and platelets in the blood.

Blood Pressure
Description: Blood pressure is the force exerted on artery walls by the heart's pumping action. Abnormal blood pressure can indicate underlying health issues.

Blood Transfusion
Description: A blood transfusion involves the transfer of blood to a patient, often necessary for individuals with anemia or blood deficiencies.

Bronchitis

Description: Bronchitis results from lung infections and requires appropriate medical treatment.

Cancer

Description: Cancer is a potentially life-threatening disease characterized by the uncontrolled growth of abnormal cells, with specific types named after their location in the body.

Catheter

Description: A catheter is a tube used to administer or withdraw fluids from the body.

CDHP (Consumer Driven Health Plan)

Description: A CDHP is a health insurance plan that may be tax-deductible and allows individuals to save on taxes while securing insurance coverage.

CSF (Cerebrospinal Fluid)

Description: CSF is the fluid that flows from the brain to the spinal cord, playing a crucial role in the nervous system.

Cirrhosis

Description: Cirrhosis is a condition where the liver shrinks and hardens, potentially impairing its function, often linked to alcoholism.

Claim
Description: A claim refers to a medical bill submitted to an insurance company in a standardized format.

Cognition
Description: Cognition encompasses higher-level brain functions, including judgment, memory, and intelligence.

Concussion
Description: A concussion is a medical condition resulting from head trauma, sometimes causing temporary unconsciousness.

CVD (Cardiovascular Disease)
Description: CVD encompasses various diseases affecting the heart and blood vessels, necessitating awareness and treatment.

Coroner
Description: A coroner investigates sudden deaths to determine the cause of death.

Delusions
Description: Delusions refer to a state of unrealistic thinking, often requiring medical attention to regain touch with reality.

Depersonalization
Description: Depersonalization involves feeling disconnected from one's environment, potentially leading to mental disorders.

Dermatitis
Description: Dermatitis is a skin disorder with multiple causes, necessitating appropriate treatment options.

Detoxification
Description: Detoxification is the process of eliminating harmful toxins and chemicals from the body using specific substances or minerals.

Diabetes
Description: Diabetes results from high blood sugar levels, often due to insulin deficiency, and requires monitoring and treatment, including dietary changes.

Dialysis

Description: Dialysis involves cleaning the blood when the kidneys fail, often achieved through a machine substituting kidney function.

Dementia

Description: Dementia is a medical condition characterized by memory loss, which can be temporary or permanent.

DME (Durable Medical Equipment)

Description: DME includes reusable physical medical equipment like wheelchairs and crutches.

Dyspnea

Description: Dyspnea refers to experiencing significant difficulty in breathing, often called shortness of breath.

ECG (Electrocardiogram)

Description: An ECG is an electronic recording of heart activity, aiding in diagnosing heart conditions.

ECT (Electroconvulsive Therapy)

Description: ECT is used for treating severe depression when other treatments are ineffective, but it can have lasting side effects.

EEG (Electroencephalogram): This medical test is performed to map brain activity, identifying various types of brain waves that can reveal information, such as the presence of seizures.

Epistaxis (Nosebleed): Epistaxis is characterized by profuse bleeding from the nose, which can result from facial injuries or occur spontaneously. Medical treatment may be necessary if the bleeding doesn't stop on its own.

Epilepsy: Epilepsy is a condition marked by unwanted electrical discharges in the brain, leading to seizures. Seizure-related body movements are involuntary.

Extubation: This is the process of removing a previously inserted tube from the lungs, which was used for oxygen delivery. The opposite procedure is called intubation.

Febrile: Febrile describes the state of having a fever.

Fistula: A fistula is an abnormal connection between two organs, often causing discomfort or pain.

Fractures: A fracture is a broken bone. A compound fracture occurs when the bone protrudes through the skin, potentially requiring an extended healing period.

Gallstones: Gallstones are stone-like formations in the gallbladder. Small stones may not necessitate surgery, but larger ones may require gallbladder removal.

Gastritis: Gastritis is the inflammation of the stomach's inner lining, often accompanied by symptoms like nausea, vomiting, burning, and pain.

Gastroenteritis: This condition results from inflammation in the stomach or intestines and can sometimes lead to infection.

Hematemesis: Hematemesis is the vomiting of blood, and its severity can indicate serious underlying issues.

Hematoma: Hematoma is a medical term for a bruise.

Hematuria: Hematuria is the presence of blood in the urine and can signal various underlying problems, such as kidney stones or infections.

Hemoglobin: Hemoglobin is a protein rich in iron found in abundance in red blood cells, primarily responsible for transporting oxygen to body tissues.

Hemoptysis: Hemoptysis is the act of coughing up blood.

Heart Disease: Any medical condition affecting the heart falls under the category of heart disease.

Hernia: Hernia is a medical condition where one body part protrudes into another, sometimes requiring surgical repair.

Hallucination: Hallucination refers to the perception of non-existent things, such as hearing voices or seeing objects that aren't real. It can occur in conditions like drug abuse and schizophrenia.

Hepatitis: Hepatitis is caused by liver inflammation, often resulting from exposure to toxic substances, alcohol, or infectious sources like shared needles or contaminated food.

Hospice: Hospice is a specialized care facility or service for individuals diagnosed with terminal illnesses, offering a supportive environment for those with limited time to live, and it can also be provided in a home setting.

Hyperglycemia
In this scenario, the blood's glucose level exceeds the typical range, often signaling the presence of diabetes.

Hypoglycemia
In this case, there is a deficit of glucose in the bloodstream.

Hypothermia
This medical condition occurs when the body temperature drops significantly. If low body temperature persists or continues to decrease, it can lead to fatality, necessitating urgent medical attention.

Incontinence
This condition arises when an individual cannot control their bladder function, and it can also extend to bowel control issues, often requiring the use of protective garments.

Infusion
Infusion refers to the gradual administration of a drug or other fluid into the body via the veins.

Insomnia
Insomnia is a state where individuals have difficulty sleeping, which can lead to various physical health problems. Sufficient sleep is essential for regular functioning, and untreated insomnia can result in issues like car accidents and high blood pressure.

Intravenous
This is a method of injecting substances or chemicals directly into the bloodstream using a needle. In specific medical cases, intravenous injections are necessary when no other route of medication administration is suitable.

Ischemia
Ischemia is the condition where blood supply to a specific area is obstructed. Depending on where this occurs, it can lead to various complications. For instance, heart ischemia can cause angina (chest pain), while untreated limb ischemia can result in tissue death or limb loss.

Jaundice
Jaundice results from an excess of bilirubin in the blood due to liver issues, causing a yellowish discoloration of the skin and eyes. It can also affect newborns.

Korsakoff's syndrome

This condition often affects individuals with a history of excessive alcohol consumption, leading to memory loss (amnesia) and confabulation (making up information to fill memory gaps).

Mantoux test
The Mantoux test is a skin test used to determine if a person has been exposed to tuberculosis (TB). It requires interpretation by a trained professional.

Migraine
Migraine is characterized by severe headaches caused by the dilation of blood vessels in the head. It can be disabling and last for days, with symptoms including headache, nausea, light sensitivity, dizziness, and fatigue.

Meningitis
Meningitis is the inflammation of the meninges, the protective covering of the brain. It is typically caused by an infection and requires immediate treatment.

Morbidity
Morbidity refers to the various outcomes that can result from a disease.

Morphine

Morphine is a common pain-relief drug that may not be effective for all types of pain, including kidney stone-related pain.

Mania
Mania is a hyperactive mental state characterized by euphoria and restlessness, often associated with bipolar disorder.

MRI
MRI scans provide images of internal organs using magnetic fields and radio waves to better understand the body's interior.

Munchausen syndrome
This psychological illness involves individuals feigning medical illnesses to gain attention, sometimes causing harm to themselves.

Neuritis
Neuritis is the painful inflammation of neural tissue.

Nebulizer
A nebulizer, powered by an air pump, converts liquid into a mist for inhalation, often used for asthma and breathing disorders.

Night sweats

Night sweats can be a sign of serious diseases like cancer or linked to conditions like menopause or thyroid issues, and they are a common symptom of tuberculosis.

Edema
Edema is the accumulation of fluids in tissues, which can lead to swelling, such as edema in the ankles and lower legs associated with heart failure.

Esophagus
The esophagus is part of the digestive tract, a muscular tube running from the mouth to the stomach, and esophageal spasms can mimic heart attack symptoms.

Palpitations
Palpitations occur when the heart beats rapidly, and while not necessarily a sign of a severe heart condition, they can be uncomfortable and should be evaluated by a medical professional.

Pancreas
The pancreas is a gland located behind the stomach responsible for insulin production and playing a role in digestion.

Paralysis

Paralysis is the inability of a part of the body to respond, often resulting from nerve damage and varying in permanence based on the cause.

Paranoia
Frequently associated with psychological disorders such as schizophrenia, this condition often results in hallucinations, delusions, and various anxieties. Paranoia can also precipitate the development of phobias and, when fear intensifies, may lead to social challenges.

PCP (Primary Care Physician)
The acronym PCP stands for the primary healthcare provider who offers initial medical care to a patient. This physician collaborates with specialists and other healthcare providers on the patient's behalf. Many health insurance companies mandate the selection of a primary care physician to oversee a patient's care.

Personality Disorder
Characterized by erratic mood swings and behaviors, personality disorders encompass conditions like borderline personality disorder, narcissistic personality disorder, and histrionic personality disorder, among others.

Pediculosis

When the skin is infested by pediculosis lice, it is colloquially known as scabies. This infestation causes intense itching and an irresistible urge to scratch. Swift treatment is crucial as it can rapidly spread over the body and to others.

Phlebitis
Phlebitis is a medical condition marked by inflammation of vein walls, which can be caused by various factors, including the initiation of an IV or the use of contaminated needles, particularly among drug addicts.

Psychosis
Individuals experiencing psychosis often exhibit impaired judgment and memory, which can lead them to commit acts they may not be aware of. Timely medical attention is crucial as this condition can deteriorate rapidly.

Psychosomatic
Referring to the connection between the mind and body, psychosomatic conditions manifest physical symptoms that are rooted in psychological stress, not due to a viral or other physiological illness.

Pulmonary
Pertaining to anything related to the respiratory system or lungs.

Pulse

A fundamental medical term denoting the rhythmic pulsation of an artery. It is one of the initial assessments performed by paramedics and doctors to evaluate a patient's condition, often measured at the wrist or neck.

Radiology

Radiology encompasses various imaging techniques, including X-rays, CT scans, and MRI scans, which utilize radiation and electromagnetic methods to produce detailed internal body images.

Rapport

In a medical context, rapport describes the empathetic relationship formed between a healthcare worker, such as a doctor or nurse, and a patient.

Resuscitation

Resuscitation involves reviving an unconscious or near-death individual, often associated with CPR (Cardiopulmonary Resuscitation) or other life-saving measures. Some individuals opt for a Do Not Resuscitate (DNR) directive.

Scabies

Scabies refers to an inflammatory skin condition caused by an infestation of pediculosis lice.

Schizophrenia
A complex mental illness typically attributed to genetic factors, schizophrenia is characterized by peculiar social behavior and the perception of unreal things.

Sepsis
Sepsis is an infection, often bacterial, that enters the bloodstream and disseminates throughout the body. A patient is termed "septic" when such an infection has become widespread, which can be life-threatening.

Shock
Medically, shock pertains to abnormally low blood pressure, often a result of sudden blood loss due to trauma, and it is an emergency condition.

Sinus
While "sinus" can have multiple meanings, it typically refers to cavities in the skull bone, particularly facial sinuses.

Spleen

An essential organ situated in the upper abdominal region, the spleen plays a crucial role in the immune system.

Sternum
The sternum is the central chest bone where the ribs meet, serving to protect the heart and lungs.

Steroid
Steroids, including anabolic steroids, are chemical compounds produced by the adrenal glands and are employed in medicine to combat inflammation. Anabolic steroids, used by athletes, serve a different purpose–building muscle and weight.

Stroke
A stroke occurs when blood flow to the brain is obstructed, often due to a blood clot, resulting in symptoms such as weakness, paralysis, and, in severe cases, death.

Syndrome
A syndrome refers to a collection of symptoms occurring simultaneously without a known cause, distinguished from a disease where a set of symptoms has a known cause or predictable course.

Tetanus

Tetanus is a bacterial infection typically triggered by puncture wounds and can be prevented through vaccination. If untreated, it can lead to fatalities.

Thiamine
Thiamine is synonymous with Vitamin B1, essential for heart and brain health. Low thiamine levels are frequently observed in individuals with alcoholism.

Tolerance
In a medical context, tolerance represents the body's adaptation to an external substance or force, requiring increasing amounts to achieve the desired effect with regular exposure.

Transference
Transference is the unconscious act of projecting one's emotions or attitudes toward another person, often observed in psychoanalysis when patients redirect past feelings onto their therapists.

Tuberculosis
Tuberculosis (TB) is a bacterial infection that can affect various body parts, with both latent and active forms. Active TB is contagious and typically spreads through respiratory droplets from coughing.

Ulcer

An ulcer is an open sore or wound that can occur on the skin or internally, commonly found on the stomach lining, skin, or cornea.

Urological
Urological pertains to anything related to the kidneys, bladder, or the urinary system.

Ventilator
A ventilator is an artificial respiratory device that assists patients in breathing by delivering air through a tube placed in the trachea, usually through the nose or mouth.

Virus
Viruses are microorganisms smaller than bacteria that require a host cell to reproduce. They can cause substantial harm to the body and are not affected by antibiotics, including well-known viruses like Ebola, HIV, and Influenza.

Wheeze
Wheezing is a breathing pattern often accompanied by a whistling sound and is commonly observed in patients with conditions like asthma or chronic obstructive lung diseases.

The world of medicine is indeed vast and ever-evolving. Understanding these fundamental medical terms is a valuable starting point for improving communication with healthcare professionals. Continually expanding your knowledge and staying informed about medical advancements will empower you to have more informed discussions with your doctor and better advocate for your health. Gaining expertise in this field may take time, but the journey of learning about your body and healthcare is a worthy endeavor.

Chapter 6

Understanding Medical Body System Terminology

In the field of medicine, it's essential for individuals involved in healthcare or receiving medical treatment to grasp the terminology used. While medical professionals are familiar with these terms, laypeople may find it challenging to comprehend the language used in medical reports. Therefore, it's advantageous to have a fundamental understanding of the human body and the terminology commonly employed to describe its various components.

Learning Medical Terminology by Categories

One approach to facilitate the learning of medical terms is by categorizing them. The human body is a complex system of interconnected organs, each working collaboratively to perform specific functions. These groups of organs are known as body systems, and each is responsible for crucial bodily functions.

Human beings typically have eight primary body systems:

The Respiratory System: Comprising the lungs, nasal passages, bronchi, pharynx, trachea, diaphragm, and bronchial tubes, this system is responsible for oxygen intake and the removal of carbon dioxide.

The Nervous System: This system includes the brain, spinal cord, nerves, eyes, nose, ears, tongue, and skin, governing bodily activities and responses to stimuli.

The Digestive System: Consisting of teeth, tongue, esophagus, stomach, pancreas, liver, and intestines, it breaks down and absorbs food for utilization.

The Excretory System: Comprised of the ureter, kidneys, bladder, and skin, this system helps regulate water and salt balance in the body.

The Endocrine System: Including the pituitary and adrenal glands, thyroid gland, and gonads, this system produces and regulates hormones.

The Skeletal and Muscular System: This system encompasses bones and muscles, governing bodily movements and providing protection.

The Circulatory System: Comprising the heart, lymph system, blood vessels, and blood, it transports nutrients, water, salts, and metabolic waste throughout the body, as well as aiding in the immune response.

The Integumentary System: This system consists of the entire body's skin, maintaining tissue moisture, regulating body temperature, and protecting against external injuries and pathogens.

As we proceed, we will focus on the terminology associated with sub-systems falling under these primary body systems. We'll also discuss the individual body parts within these systems and their respective functions.

Additional Body Systems and Terminology

In addition to the primary body systems, there are additional systems and related terminology to understand:

Appendicular Skeleton: Comprising 126 bones in the upper and lower limbs, as well as the pectoral and pelvic girdles, this system enables movement and provides protection for reproductive, digestive, and urinary systems.

Carpel: A system consisting of eight small wrist bones, derived from the Latin word "carpus."

Cervical Spine: Comprising seven bony rings in the neck, these vertebrae support the head, protect the spinal cord, and facilitate head and neck mobility.

Coccyx: A triangular bone at the bottom of the spine, also known as the tailbone.

Diarthrosis: A freely moving joint enclosed within one articular capsule.

Femoral Neck: The upper section of the femur connecting the head to the shaft.

Femur: The thighbone, forming joints at the hip and knee.

Fibula: The smaller of two leg bones, running parallel to the tibia from the knee to the ankle.

Humerus: The bone in the upper arm, forming the shoulder and elbow joints.

Lumbar Spine: Comprising five vertebral bodies, these stack on top of each other with discs in between, running from the lower thoracic spine to the sacrum.

Metacarpal: Each of the five hand bones.

Metatarsal: Each of the foot bones.

Olecranon: The bony part that gives the elbow prominence, forming the end of the ulna in the forearm.

Patella: The kneecap.

Pelvic Girdle: The structure formed by the pelvis, providing an attachment area for pelvic fins.

Phalanges: The bones of fingers and toes, also referred to as phalanx.

Radius: The shorter, thicker bone in the forearm, aligned to the thumb side.

Ribs: Twelve slender, curved bones articulating to the spine in pairs, protecting the thoracic cavity and its organs. They make up the thoracic skeleton, with seven pairs along the front and back and three attached to the posterior, two of them appearing incomplete.

Sacrum

The sacrum consists of fused vertebrae and typically resides in the lower region of the lumbar spine. It comprises a flat, triangular bone situated in the lower back, positioned between the hipbones within the pelvis.

Shoulder Girdle

The shoulder girdle, also known as the pectoral girdle, is composed of two bones, the clavicle and the scapula, linking the human arm to the axial skeleton.

Sternum

The sternum is the primary component of the breastbone.

Tarsal

The tarsal is a bone located within the tarsus, a cluster of small bones that together make up a significant portion of the hind limb. The human tarsus is composed of seven bones, which form the ankle and the upper part of the foot. These bones include three cuneiform bones, the talus, the cuboid, the calcaneus, and the navicular.

Thoracic Spine

The thoracic spine is the central segment of the spine, situated just below the cervical spine. It consists of twelve vertebral bodies and has a somewhat C-shaped structure.

Tibia

The tibia is positioned between the knee and ankle in the lower leg and is one of the two major bones in this area. It lies beneath the other bone, the fibula, and is the larger of the two, running parallel to it.

Ulna

The ulna is one of the two bones that comprise the main part of the forearm, being the thinner and longer of the two, situated on the opposite side of the thumb.

Chapter 7

The Creation of Plurals in Medical Terminology

Within the realm of medical language, the formation of plurals does not adhere to the typical rules of standard English. In the medical context, it is essential to recognize and follow the unique pluralization rules that apply. Thus, it is crucial to familiarize oneself with the specific regulations governing the transition from singular to plural forms within the medical field. Nevertheless, similar to standard English, there exist exceptions where certain words do not conform to established rules and must be memorized individually.

Here are various categories of pluralization rules:

Medical terms ending with -a:

Singular words ending in 'a' change to 'ae' in their plural form. For instance, "vertebra" becomes "vertebrae," and "pleura" becomes "pleurae."

Medical terms ending with -is:

Words ending in 'is' in the singular form replace it with 'es' to form their plural, such as "arthrosis" becoming "arthroses" and "diagnosis" becoming "diagnoses."

Medical terms ending with -ix or -ex:

Singular terms ending in 'ix' or 'ex' transform to 'ices' in their plural form, like "appendix" becoming "appendices" and "fornix" becoming "fornices."

Medical terms ending with -itis:

Words ending with 'itis' in singular change to 'itides' in plural. For example, "arthritis" becomes "athritides," and "hepatitis" becomes "hepatites."

Medical terms ending with -nx:

Terms concluding with 'nx' change to 'nges' in the plural form. For instance, "phalanx" becomes "phalanges," and "larynx" becomes "larynges."

Medical terms ending with -um:

Words ending in 'um' drop it and take up 'a' to create their plurals, as in "endocardium" becoming "endocardia" and "myocardium" becoming "myocardia."

Medical terms ending with -us:

Terms ending in 'us' in the singular form change to 'i' in their plural form. For instance, "digitus" becomes "digiti" and "oesophagus" becomes "oesophagi."

Medical terms ending with -y:

Singular terms ending in 'y' become plurals by dropping 'y' and adding 'ies.' For example, "therapy" becomes "therapies" and "cardiomyopathy" becomes "cardiomyopathies."

Medical terms ending with -ion:

Words ending in 'ion' in singular simply add an 's' to form the plural, such as "chorion" becoming "chorions."

Medical terms ending with -ma or -oma:

Terms ending in 'ma' or 'oma' in singular add 'ta' to form their plural, like "carcinoma" becoming "carcinomata" and "leiomyoma" becoming "leiomyomata."

Medical terms ending with -yx, -ax, or -ix:

These terms change in plural by replacing the 'x' at the end with 'c' and then adding 'es,' such as "appendix" becoming "appendices" and "calyx" becoming "calyces."

Unconventional plurals:

Some medical terms do not follow any specific pattern, and their plurals must be learned individually.
For example, "vas" becomes "vasa," "pons" becomes "pontes," "femur" becomes "femora," and so on.

It's essential to note that proper understanding and application of these rules are crucial when working with medical terminology.

Chapter 8

Acronyms, Homonyms, and Eponyms

Acronyms, which consist of letter combinations at the start of specific words, are pronounced as independent words. Examples of commonly used acronyms in everyday life include "UNEP" for the United Nations Environment Program and "ISO" for the International Standards Organization. Similarly, in the medical field, there are abbreviations for long medical terms with two or more words.

Here is a list of medical acronyms:

AAA: Abdominal Aortic Aneurysm
AAS: Acute Abdominal Series

ABD: Abdomen

ABG: Arterial Blood Gas

AC: Before eating

ACLS: Advanced Cardiac Life Support

ACTH: Adrenocorticotropic Hormone

AD: Autonomic Dysreflexia

Ad lib: An unrestricted amount, e.g., "feeding without restriction."

ADH: Anti-Diuretic Hormone

ADL: Activities of Daily Living

AF: Atrial Fibrillation or Afebrile

AFB: Acid-Fast Bacilli

AFP: Alpha-Fetoprotein

AFO: Ankle Foot Orthosis

A/G: Albumin/Globulin ratio

AI: Aortic Insufficiency

AKA: Above The Knee Amputation

ALL: Acute Lymphocytic Leukemia

ALS: Amyotrophic Lateral Sclerosis (also known as Lou Gehrig's disease)

Amb: Ambulate

AML: Acute Myelogenous Leukemia

ANA: Antinuclear Antibody

AOB: Alcohol On Breath

AODM: Adult Onset Diabetes Mellitus

AP: Anteroposterior or Abdominal Perineal

ARDS: Acute Respiratory Distress Syndrome

ARF: Acute Renal Failure

AS: Aortic Stenosis

ASAP: As Soon As Possible

ASCVD: Atherosclerotic Cardiovascular Disease

ASD: Atrial Septal Defect

ASHD: Atherosclerotic Heart Disease

ASIA: American Spinal Injury Association

AV: Atrioventricular

A-V: Arteriovenous

A-VO2: Arteriovenous Oxygen

BBB: Bundle Branch Block

BC: Bowel Care

BCAA: Branched Chain Amino Acids

BE: Barium Enema

BEE: Basal Energy Expenditure

Bid: Twice a day

Bilat: Bilateral

BKA: Below The Knee Amputation

BM: Bone Marrow or Bowel Movement

BMR: Basal Metabolic Rate

BOM: Bilateral Otitis Media

BP: Blood Pressure

BPH: Benign Prostatic Hypertrophy

BPM: Beats Per Minute

BRBPR: Bright Red Blood Per Rectum

BRP: Bathroom Privileges

BS: Bowel or Breath Sounds

BUN: Blood Urea Nitrogen

BW: Body Weight

BX: Biopsy

C&S: Culture And Sensitivity

CA: Cancer

Ca: Calcium

CAA: Crystalline Amino Acids

CABG: Coronary Artery Bypass Graft

CAD: Coronary Artery Disease

CAT: Computerized Axial Tomography

CBC: Complete Blood Count

CBG: Capillary Blood Gas

CC: Chief Complaint

CCU: Clean Catch Urine or Cardiac Care Unit

CCV: Critical Closing Volume

CF: Cystic Fibrosis

CGL: Chronic Granulocytic Leukemia

CHF: Congestive Heart Failure

CHO: Carbohydrate

CI: Cardiac Index

CML: Chronic Myelogenous Leukemia

CMV: Cytomegalovirus

CN: Cranial Nerves

CNS: Central Nervous System

CO: Cardiac Output

C/O: Complaining Of

COLD: Chronic Obstructive Lung Disease

COPD: Chronic Obstructive Pulmonary Disease

CP: Chest Pain or Cerebral Palsy

CPAP: Continuous Positive Airway Pressure

CPK: Creatinine Phosphokinase

CPR: Cardiopulmonary Resuscitation

CRCL: Creatinine Clearance

CRF: Chronic Renal Failure

CRP: C-reactive protein

CRTS is an abbreviation for Certified Recreational Therapy Specialist.

CSF is short for Cerebrospinal Fluid.

CT stands for Computerized Tomography.

CVA is an abbreviation for Cerebrovascular Accident, and it is sometimes used to refer to Costovertebral Angle.

CVAT is an acronym for CVA Tenderness.

CXR is an abbreviation that stands for Chest X-Ray.

In the medical field, **DC** is an abbreviation for discontinue, and it is also sometimes used to mean discharge.

In the medical language, **D&C** is an abbreviation for Dilation And Curettage.

DDx is used in the medical field to stand for Differential Diagnosis.

In the medical field, **D5W** is an abbreviation for 5% Dextrose In Water.

DI is an abbreviation for Diabetes Insipidus.

DIC is an abbreviation for Disseminated Intravascular Coagulopathy.

DIP is an abbreviation for Distal Interphalangeal Joint.

DJD is an abbreviation for Degenerative Joint Disease.

DKA is an abbreviation for Diabetic Ketoacidosis.

DM is an abbreviation for Diabetes Mellitus.

DNA stands for Deoxyribonucleic Acid.

In the medical field, **DOA** is an abbreviation for Dead On Arrival.

DOE is an abbreviation for dyspnea on exertion.

DPL is used in the medical field as an abbreviation for Diagnostic Peritoneal Lavage.

DPT is used as an abbreviation for Diphtheria, Pertussis, Tetanus.

DVT is an abbreviation for Deep Venous Thrombosis.

DX is used as an abbreviation for diagnosis.

EAA is an abbreviation for Essential Amino Acids.

ECD is an abbreviation for External Continence Device.

ECG is an abbreviation for electrocardiogram.
ECT is an abbreviation for Electroconvulsive Therapy.

ED is an abbreviation for Erectile Dysfunction.

EFAD is used as an abbreviation for Essential Fatty Acid Deficiency.

EMG is an abbreviation for Electromyogram.

EMV is an abbreviation for Eyes, Motor, Verbal response.

ENT is used in the medical field as an abbreviation for Ears, Nose, And Throat.

EOM is an abbreviation for Extraocular Muscles.

ET is used in the medical field as an abbreviation for Endotracheal.

ETT is an abbreviation for Endotracheal Tube.

ERCP is an abbreviation for Endoscopic Retrograde Cholangio–Pancreatography.
ETOH, in the medical field, is an abbreviation for ethanol.

EUA is an abbreviation for examination under anesthesia.

Homonyms, in a general sense, are words that share the same pronunciation but have different meanings, often with varying spellings. Some familiar homonyms in everyday language include "feet" and "feat," "meat" and "meet," "bear" and "bare," and others.

Here are homonyms commonly used in the medical field:

"Ileum" versus "ilium": "Ileum" refers to a part of the colon, while "ilium" is a pelvic bone portion.
"Lice" and "lyse": "Lice" are parasites, and "lyse" means to destroy cells by using lysins.
"Loop" and "Loupe": "Loop" is a circular-shaped ring, and "loupe" is a type of magnifying glass.
"Mnemo" and "Pneumo": "Mnemo" relates to memory, and "pneumo" indicates a connection to the lungs.

"Mucus" and "Mucous": "Mucus" refers to secretions produced by mucous membranes, while "mucous" is an adjective describing something that looks like mucus.

"Plane" and "plain": In the medical field, "plane" indicates an anatomical level, while "plain" means something uncomplicated or not fancy, like plain X-rays.

"Plural" and "Pleural": "Plural" means more than one, while "pleural" is related to things pertaining to the lungs.

"Radical" and "radical": "Radical" means drastic, while "radical" means the smallest branch emerging from a blood vessel.

Eponyms are names given to various things in the medical field based on historical significance. This can include diseases named after the scientist or doctor who discovered them, as well as treatments named after individuals who made them prominent. While modern practice tends to be more descriptive, existing eponyms remain unchanged and important to know.

Here are some common eponyms in the medical field:

"Parkinson's disease" is named after James Parkinson, an Englishman who wrote about it in 1817.

"Alzheimer's" is named after Alois Alzheimer, a Bavarian psychiatrist and pathologist.

"Hashimoto's disease" is named after Hakaru Hashimoto, a Japanese doctor who wrote a report in 1912.

"Crohn's disease" is named after Burrill Crohn, an American gastroenterologist.

These eponyms are important to recognize in the medical field due to their historical significance.

Chapter 9

Medical Terminology for Body Structures

In the healthcare sector, it's essential to understand not only the organs comprising the body's systems but also a wide range of terminology. These terms encompass descriptions of organ proximity, organ function (both normal and abnormal), organ position, and other medical conditions affecting various body parts.

Here are some medical terms related to the human body's structure:

Prefix "ab-":

This prefix is employed in various contexts to indicate moving away from a specific body part or being apart from it.

For example:
Abduction: This term is used to describe the movement of a limb away from the body's central axis.
Abnormal: A frequently used term to signify a deviation from the normal state.

Abbreviation "Abd":

In the medical field, "Abd" is an abbreviation for the abdomen.
Terms "Abdomin" or "Abdomino":

These terms simply refer to the abdomen.

Term "Abdominal":

In medical terminology, "abdominal" describes anything related to the abdomen.

Term "Abdominopelvic":

This term is used to describe a body cavity encompassing both the abdominal and pelvic cavities. Organs contained within this large cavity include a significant portion of the small and large intestines, the liver, pancreas, spleen, stomach, kidneys, and gallbladder.

Term "Abduction":

Signifies the movement away from the body's central axis.

Term "Adduction":

Refers to the act of moving toward the body's central axis.

Term "Adhesion":

In the medical context, adhesion refers to the formation of scar tissue that binds anatomical surfaces that are typically separate.

Suffixes for Adjectives (ac/al/ar/ary/eal/ic/iac/ior/ous/tic):

These suffixes are used to create adjectives indicating a relationship to something.

For example:

Abdominal	Myalgia	Perineal	Corneal	Biliary tract
Bacteriocidal	Oesophageal	Hematotic	Hepatic artery	Femoral

Ad and Ad-

In a medical context, the prefix and suffix "ad" convey the notion of moving or directing toward a specific point. For instance:

"Medi-ad" implies movement toward the center or middle.

"Ad-duction" denotes the action of moving a body part toward the central region of the main body.

Anastomosis
Anastomosis refers to the surgical connection of two blood vessels or ducts, enabling the unrestricted flow of blood or other substances from one side to the other. This term is also employed when linking different segments of the bowel to facilitate the smooth passage of bowel contents.

Anatomical Position
This term describes the standard standing posture in which the entire body is upright, the head faces upward, arms rest at the sides with palms forward, and the legs are parallel while the feet are slightly apart with toes pointing forward.

Ant
In the medical field, "ant" is an abbreviation for "anterior."

Anter/ior
This term signifies the position of a body structure
or organ when it is situated on the front side of the
body.

Anter/o
This term references the front of the body, with
"anterior" sometimes serving as a synonym.

AP
In the medical context, "AP" stands for
"anteroposterior."

Back
In medical terminology, "back" refers to the
posterior side of the body or the rear.

Bx
"Bx" is used as an abbreviation for "biopsy."

Cartilage
Cartilage is a term that describes the ribs.

Caud(ad): This term is employed to describe the
direction towards the tail or the posterior. An
adjective derived from this term is "caudally."

Caudo: Caudo represents the tail or the lower part of the human body, often used as a prefix or suffix. For example, "Caudofemoralis" refers to a muscle in the pelvic limb, derived from the Latin word "cauda," meaning thighbone.

Craniocaudal: This term indicates the direction of an X-ray beam passing through the body. In medical context, the point of entry of the X-ray beam is the cranial end, while the exit point is the caudal end.

Cauterize: This term is used to denote the process of burning abnormal tissue using methods like heat, electricity, or chemicals, including silver nitrate. At times, abnormal tissue is eliminated by freezing.

Cephal(o): This term pertains to the head, and from it, "cephalad" is derived, meaning towards the head.

Cervic(o): This term refers to the human neck and gives rise to related terms like "cervix uteri," denoting the neck of the uterus.

Cervical: "Cervical" describes what is related to the human neck or the neck of the uterus.

Chondr(o): This term signifies cartilage, originating from the Greek word "chondros."

Chondr/oma: This refers to a mass of cartilage cells that can resemble a tumor, sometimes growing on cartilage surfaces or emerging from the medullary cavity's cartilage.

CT: CT stands for computed tomography.

Crani(o): This term is used to denote the human skull, also known as the cranium.

Cranial: "Cranial" signifies that which relates to the human skull or cranium.

CXR: CXR is an abbreviation for "chest X-ray," and it can also mean "chest radiograph."

Cyt(o): This term represents a cell and is often used as a prefix in words like "cytoplasm" and "cytokinesis."

Cytology: In medicine, "cytology" is the study of human cells.

Cyt-o-lysis: This term refers to cell separation, dissolution, or destruction, combining "cyto" (cell) and "-lysis" (loosening or destruction).

Cyt/o/meter: This is the name for an instrument used to count or measure cells, typically a glass chamber or slide with known volume.

Cyto-toxic: "Cyto-toxic" describes a substance capable of destroying cells, with "cyto" relating to cells and "toxic" to poison.

Dist/al: This term indicates a point far from the central area or the main body, in contrast to "proximal," which means close to the body's center.

Dist(o): "Dist(o)" signifies far or farthest.

Doppler
This pertains to technology that operates with ultrasonic waves to generate audible sounds of blood flow within arteries. It's commonly known as Doppler technology.

Dors(al)
This indicates a relation to the posterior or back of the body. For example, one can mention the dorsal view.

Dors(o)
This term describes the back of the human body and is often used as a prefix. An instance is "dorsolateral," which means relating to the back.

Endoscopy
This involves using an endoscope, a specialized illuminated instrument, to visually inspect the interior of an organ or cavity.

Epigastric region
This denotes the area above or on the stomach.

Fluoroscopy
It's a radiographic procedure that visualizes internal organ movement using X-ray imaging with a fluorescent screen, creating detailed internal images.

Frontal plane
This term is synonymous with the coronal plane. It refers to the section dividing the body into front (anterior) and back (posterior) parts, or ventral and dorsal, respectively.

Gastr(o)
This relates to the stomach.

Gastric
Gastric signifies something related to the stomach.

Inguin(o)
This term refers to the groin.

Inguinal
Inguinal indicates a connection with the groin.

Hist(o)
This term relates to body tissue and is often used as a prefix to denote tissue-related matters.

Histologist
A histologist is an expert in the study of body tissue.

Traverse plane
This phrase denotes a horizontal or cross-sectional plane that divides the body into upper (superior) and lower (inferior) sections.

Hypochondriac region
This region lies immediately below a person's ribs.

Hypogastric region
This term refers to the area immediately below a person's stomach.

Ili(o)

This term is used for the ilium or flank and is often employed in forming compound words related to the ileum.

Here is a perfect example:

iliofemoral	iliocostal	iliocostalis	Iliocaudal	iliopagus
iliothoracopagus	ilioxiphopagus	iliolumbar	iliocolotomy	iliococcygeal

Iliac

In the medical context, this term is employed to indicate a relation to the ilium bone.

Ilium

Referring to the upper section of the hipbone, it also denotes the region within the abdomen extending from the end of the ribs to the groin or pubic area.

Infer(ior)

A term within the medical field signifying a location situated below or towards the end or tail.

Infer(o)

This term simply means a location beneath or lower than another.

Inflammation

Describes the body's protective response when exposed to allergens, irritants, or infections.

Inguin(o)

Used to reference the groin area.

Lat

In medical terminology, "Lat" is an abbreviation for "lateral."

Lateral
Signifies something related to or associated with the side.

Later(o)

This term indicates leaning towards one side and is sometimes used to refer to the side.

LLQ

In the medical field, "LLQ" stands for "Left Lower Quadrant."

Lumb(o)

The term "lumb" or sometimes "lumbo" is used to describe the loins or lower back.

Lumbar

Another medical term indicating a relation to the loins or lower back.

The lumbar region

Denotes the area of the human body just below the loins or lower back.

LUQ

These letters represent an abbreviation for "Left Upper Quadrant."

MRI

An abbreviation for "Magnetic Resonance Imaging."

Medi(ad)

This term refers to an area situated toward the center or middle and is often used to form words denoting a middle position, such as "median," "medium," "mediator," and similar terms.

Medi(al)

Used to denote something related to the center or middle.

Medi(o)

This term means "middle" and is often used to create other medical terminology, such as "mediotarsal."

Median plane

The median plane, also known as the midsagittal plane, is the area that symmetrically divides the human body from top to bottom, resulting in two equal and similar left and right sides.

Nucle(ar)

This term indicates an association with the nucleus.

Nucle(o)

Refers to the nucleus, a spheroid body found inside a cell, enclosed within a double membrane known as the nuclear envelope. Everything contained in this structure, including chromosomes, is referred to as nucleoplasm.

Nuclear scan

This diagnostic technique involves introducing radiopharmaceuticals into the body via ingestion, inhalation, or injection, followed by imaging the targeted organ or body part to record the concentration of the radiopharmaceutical.

PA

This can be utilized as an abbreviation with multiple medical meanings, including pernicious anemia, posteroanterior, pulmonary artery, or Physician Assistant.

"Pelv(i)" can be interchanged with **"pelv(o),"** both signifying the pelvis.

A **"pelvimeter"** is a medical instrument employed for measuring pelvis size.

"Periumbilical" is a term describing something pertaining to the area near the umbilicus.

"PET" is the acronym for Positron Emission Tomography, a radiographic technique combining computed tomography and pharmaceuticals to visualize metabolic activity in the body.

"Poster(ior)" is used to denote something related to the rear part of the body, sometimes referred to as the caudal end.

"Proxim/o" signifies an area near the body's center or close to a reference point.

"Radiography" is the process of using ionizing radiation to produce shadow images on photographic film by passing it through the body.

"Radiopharmaceutical" refers to a medication containing radioactive material used for imaging and scanning specific body parts.

"RLQ" stands for Right Lower Quadrant.

"Scan" is a medical technique for recording and displaying images of body parts or systems.

"Sepsis" describes the body's inflammatory response to infection, often accompanied by fever, low blood pressure, elevated heart rate, and increased respiratory rate.

"SPECT" stands for Single Photon Emission Computed Tomography, a nuclear imaging technique using a specialized gamma camera to create 3D images of organs.

"SPECT" is a medical abbreviation for Single Photon Emission Computed Tomography.

Spin(o):
In the medical field, the term "Spin(o)" is utilized to describe the spinal column of the human body.

Spinal:
The term "Spinal" is employed to denote something related to the spine or the spinal column in general.

Super(o):

This term signifies the upper part or a region situated above.

Superior:
"Superior" is employed to signify something at a higher level or above another in comparison. It is also used at times to denote proximity to the head.

Thorac(o):
In medical terminology, this term is used to refer to the chest.
Thoracic:
"Thoracic" is used in the medical field to indicate something associated with the chest.

Tomography:
Tomography refers to a radiographic technique that displays a detailed cross-section of body tissue or a predetermined depth of a body part. This technique creates a cross-sectional image of body organs by producing a film.

U & L:
These letters are employed as medical abbreviations, signifying Upper and Lower. Occasionally, you may see the same abbreviation written as U/L.

Ultrasonography:

This term is used to describe the medical imaging technique that produces high-quality images of the inside of body organs or tissues. The technique employs ultrasound, a mass of high-frequency sound waves that bounce off the body to generate the required images.

Umbilic(o):
This term simply means "navel," and at times, "umbilicus" is used interchangeably.

Umbilical region:
The umbilical region is the area of the human body close to the navel.

US:
This abbreviation represents "ultrasound," and sometimes it also stands for "ultrasonography."

Ventr(o):
"Ventr(o)" is a medical term used to mean the belly or the side of the abdomen.

Ventral:
This term is used to indicate that something has an association with the abdomen or the belly.

Final Thought

Congratulations on completing this medical guide! Medical terminology can pose challenges, but in this guide, we've made a diligent effort to incorporate essential information, allowing you to familiarize yourself with common medical terms.

We are confident that, using our recommended approach, you can now effortlessly decipher any medical term. Remember to retain the root words, prefixes, and suffixes we've shared to stay up-to-date.

We've also compiled a comprehensive list of frequently used medical terms, encompassing details related to radiology, insurance terminology, anatomy, diseases, and other widely employed terms. You may have encountered some of these terms previously, but now that you understand their meanings, you can employ them appropriately.

Medical science has made significant progress in recent years, and to stay current with industry standards, you must grasp these terms. This educational book is your key to comprehending your body and various medical terms accurately. It will facilitate effective communication with your healthcare provider and allow you to impress those around you with your knowledge.

You can further enhance your skills and knowledge through ongoing education and reading. Prioritize your health and well-being, and stay safe and fit!

Made in the USA
Coppell, TX
17 May 2025

49516597R00066